Ameni JERBI

Immunological investigation of autoimmune bullous dermatoses

AF534708

Ameni JERBI

Immunological investigation of autoimmune bullous dermatoses

Interest of direct immunofluorescence on skin biopsy in the exploration of autoimmune bullous dermatoses

ScienciaScripts

Imprint
Any brand names and product names mentioned in this book are subject to trademark, brand or patent protection and are trademarks or registered trademarks of their respective holders. The use of brand names, product names, common names, trade names, product descriptions etc. even without a particular marking in this work is in no way to be construed to mean that such names may be regarded as unrestricted in respect of trademark and brand protection legislation and could thus be used by anyone.

Cover image: www.ingimage.com

This book is a translation from the original published under ISBN 978-620-6-71460-6.

Publisher:
Sciencia Scripts
is a trademark of
Dodo Books Indian Ocean Ltd. and OmniScriptum S.R.L publishing group

120 High Road, East Finchley, London, N2 9ED, United Kingdom
Str. Armeneasca 28/1, office 1, Chisinau MD-2012, Republic of Moldova, Europe
Printed at: see last page
ISBN: 978-620-8-18787-3

Copyright © Ameni JERBI
Copyright © 2024 Dodo Books Indian Ocean Ltd. and OmniScriptum S.R.L publishing group

Contents

List of abbreviations

MAI: Maladies Auto-Immunes

Ag: Antigen

DBAI: Dermatoses Bulleuses Auto-Immunes. Auto-

Ac: Auto-antibodies.

JDE: Dermo-epidermal junction.

IFD: Immunofluorescence

Ac: Antibody

CHU: Centre Hospitalier Universitaire

Ig: Immunoglobulin.

C: Complement.

FITC: Fluorescein Iso Thio Cyanate.

PBS: Phosphate Buffered Saline.

Introduction

Autoimmune diseases (AIDs) are characterized by a breakdown in tolerance to the self, leading to the development of a humoral and/or cellular immune response against one or more self or autoAg antigens (Ag). This immune response is directly responsible for the tissue damage observed and the clinical manifestations associated with the disease. The body's components are then attacked by the immune system (1).

Classically, a distinction is made between organ-specific IMAs, where the immune response is directed against a particular organ, and non-organ-specific IMAs, where the immune response is directed against several organs at once.

Autoimmune bullous dermatoses (ABDs) are skin- and mucosa-specific ABDs. They are characterized by the presence of autoantibodies (auto-Ab) directed against skin and mucous membrane adhesion molecules, leading to altered function of their antigenic targets, resulting in clinical bullae and/or erosions (2,3).

Depending on the cleavage site, a distinction is made between :

- **Intraepidermal DBAI**, or the pemphigus group, is characterized by auto-Ac directed against the structural proteins of desmosomes, which ensure the cohesion of epidermal keratinocytes. Alteration of intercellular cohesion leads to the formation of intra-epidermal bubbles.
- **Subepidermal DBAI** is characterized by the presence of auto-Ac directed against components of the dermal-epidermal junction (DEJ) (hemidesmosome)(2,3).loss of dermal-epidermal adhesion leads to the formation of subepidermal bullae.

The diagnosis of DBAI is based on clinical (presence of bullae and/or cutaneous and/or mucous erosions), histopathological (evidence of intra- or sub-epidermal cleavage) and immunological (evidence of circulating or tissue-deposited auto-Ac) criteria(4).

Direct immunofluorescence (DIF) is an immunological technique performed on cryosections of peri-lesional biopsies, based on the detection of Ac deposits and/or complement fractions using specific fluorescein-conjugated Ac (2,5).

The objectives of our work were:

- Describe the results observed at the IFD in the different DBAI in 1er time.
- And to study the contribution of this technique to the diagnosis of sub- and intra-epidermal DBAI in the immunology laboratory of the CHU Habib Bourguiba in Sfax.

Materials and methods

1. Patient recruitment

This ... is a retrospective descriptive study ofskin biopsy specimens received at the immunology laboratory of CHU Habib Bourguiba Sfax for suspected DBAI between January 2018 and March 2022.

Samples were sent by the hospital departments of CHU Habib Bourguiba and CHU Hedi Chaker, private laboratories and outlying clinics in the region.

Data on epidemiological characteristics, clinical signs and suspected diagnoses were collected.

All biopsies that could not be read were excluded from this study.

2. Methods

2.1. Skin biopsies 2.1.1 Pre-analytical stage

In cases of suspected DBAI, two skin biopsies were taken for each patient, one for anatomopathological study, the other for immunological study. Biopsies for IFD are taken from peri-lesional skin, usually healthy skin. Samples are rapidly transported at room temperature in a bottle containing physiological saline **(Figure 1A)**. Contamination of the biopsy with formalin must be avoided. Once received, they are stored at -20°C until use.

2.1.2 Cryostat sectioning

Tissue sections are taken from skin biopsies using a cryostat (Leika®):

-Biopsies are oriented and fixed with a cryostat embedding gel **(Figure 1B)** on the support at a temperature of 50°C, while avoiding the formation of air bubbles **(Figure 1C)**.

-After freezing, the biopsies are sectioned at a thickness of 4 µm at the cryo-bar at -21°C **(Figure 1D)**. The cryo-sections are fixed on slides at a rate of 3 sections per slide. For each biopsy, 4 slides are prepared **(Figure 1E)**. The temperature variation between the cryostat enclosure and ambient temperature (from -21°C to
+25°C) ensures fabric fixation.

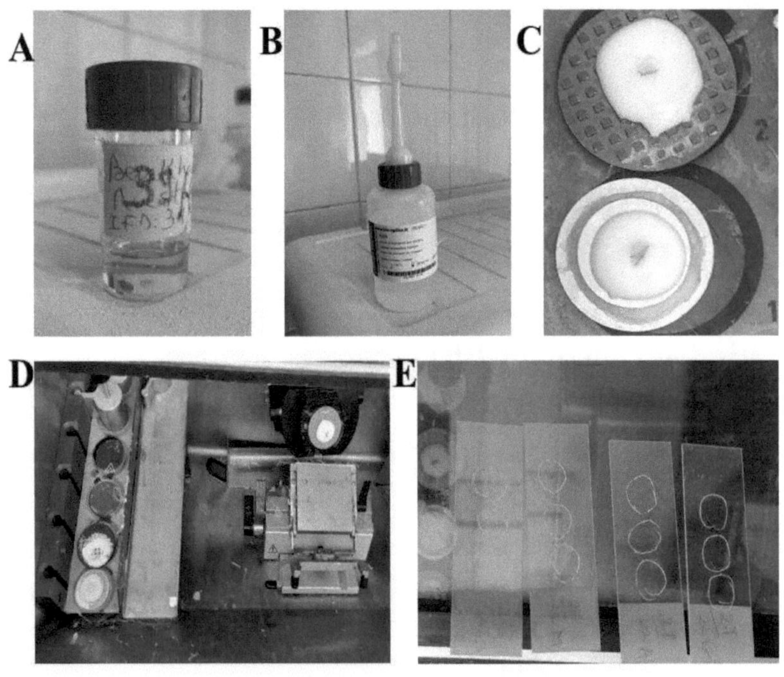

Figure1:Cutting skin tissue with a cryostat:

(A) Saline flask into which the skin biopsy is transferred; **(B)** Cryostat embedding gel;**(C)** Fixation of a biopsy on the support; **(D)**Sectioning of 4 µm thick biopsies; **(E)** Preparation of slides (4 slides for each biopsy)

2.2. Direct immunofluorescence

2.2.1.Principle

IFD is a single-step labeling technique for the detection of immunoglobulins/immune complexes (IgG, IgA and IgM) and complement fractions (C3) in tissues, using specific Ac (polyclonal anti-human Ig) (IgG, IgA, IgM, C3) conjugated to a fluorochrome. Fluorescein isothiocyanate (FITC), the most commonly used fluorochrome, produces green fluorescence when excited by blue light. It is read under a fluorescence microscope **(Figure 2)**.

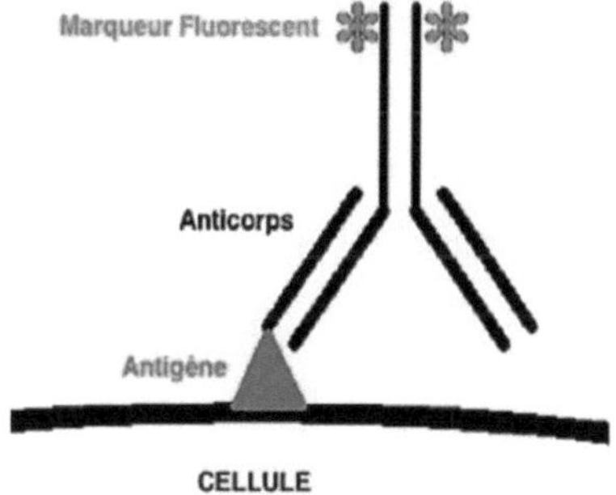

Figure 2: Principle of direct immunofluorescence

2.2.2. How it works

Each patient's slides are placed in a humidity chamber; each slide is used to add one type of labeled Ac (anti-IgG, anti-IgA, anti-IgM and anti-C3) (Euroimmun).®

Thirty microliters of Ac are added and incubated for 30 min in the dark. The slides are rinsed and immersed 2 times in PBS buffer. A third 10-minute wash is performed in a tray to which a few drops of Evans blue are added. The final step is to mount the slides with glycerol, which helps to maintain and preserve the sample.

2.2.3. Reading

Reading is done using a fluorescence microscope, at low magnification to locate the biopsy, then at high magnification (x400 objective) to note the aspects.

First of all, the quality of the cuts is assessed: the cohesion between dermis and epidermis is checked.

A biopsy is considered negative when there is no specific fluorescence in the epidermis or at the dermal-epidermal junction (DEJ). Non-specific auto-fluorescence may be observed in the dermis.

Positivity translates into specific fluorescence in the epidermis (net-like appearance) for the intra-epidermal DBAI group, or in the JDE for the sub-epidermal DBAI group.

2.3. Statistical analysis

The data collected was analyzed using Microsoft Excel.

Results

Descriptive study

Of the 770 biopsies received during the study period, we excluded biopsies that were uninterpretable or those sent in the context of pathologies other than DBAI. We included 334 biopsies **(Figure 3)**.

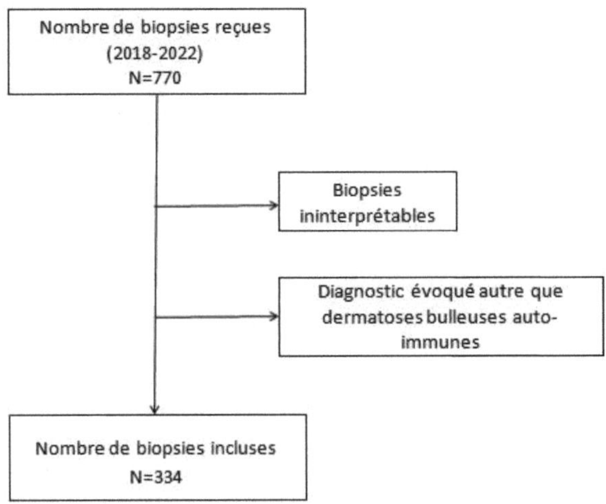

Figure 3: Selection criteria for biopsies included in our study

1.1. Epidemiological characteristics

1.1.1.Age

The average age of patients was 56.4 years, with extremes ranging from 2 to 99 years.

The age group most affected was over 70 (32% of cases) **(Figure 4)**.

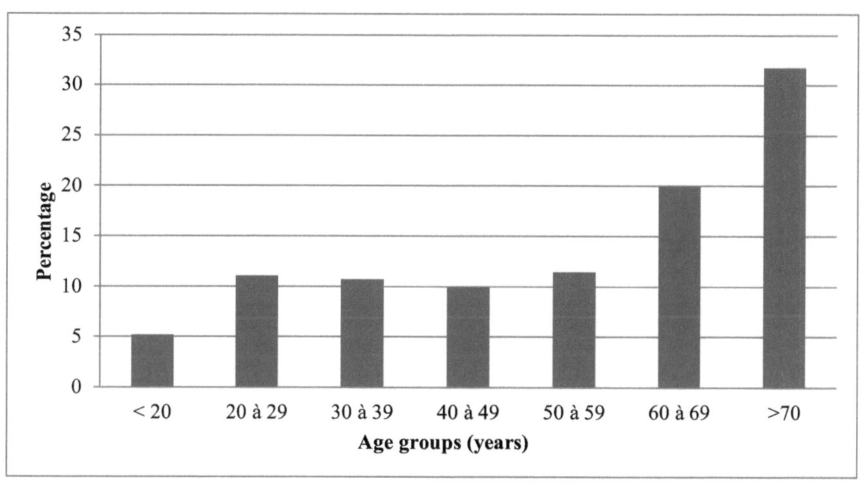

Figure 4: Age distribution of patients

Subepidermal DBAI seems to affect older subjects, with a peak in patients aged over 70. Intra-epidermal DBAI, on the other hand, mainly affects young adults, with a peak in patients aged between 40 and 49. The distribution of diagnoses by age group is **shown in figure 5**.

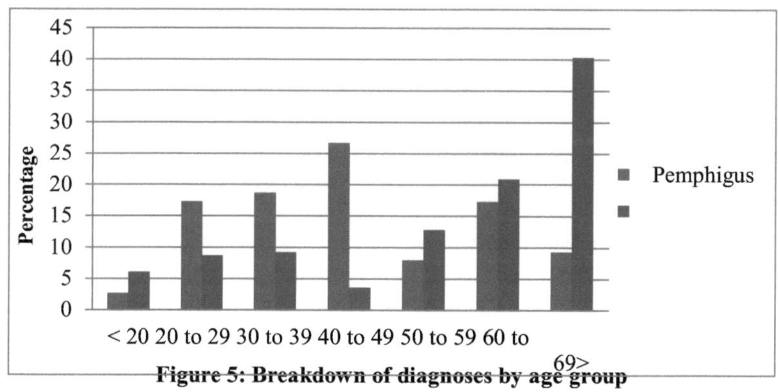

Figure 5: Breakdown of diagnoses by age group

1.1.2. Gender

The overall distribution of patients by gender revealed a predominance of females, with an F/H sex ratio of 1.7 **(Figure 6)**.

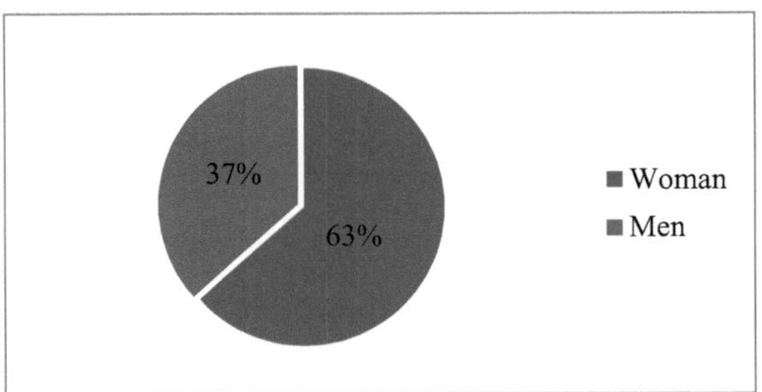

Figure 6: Distribution of patients by gender

The most affected population was female, for both intra-epidermal and sub-epidermal DBAI, with rates of 74.5% and 59.2% respectively **(Figure 7).**

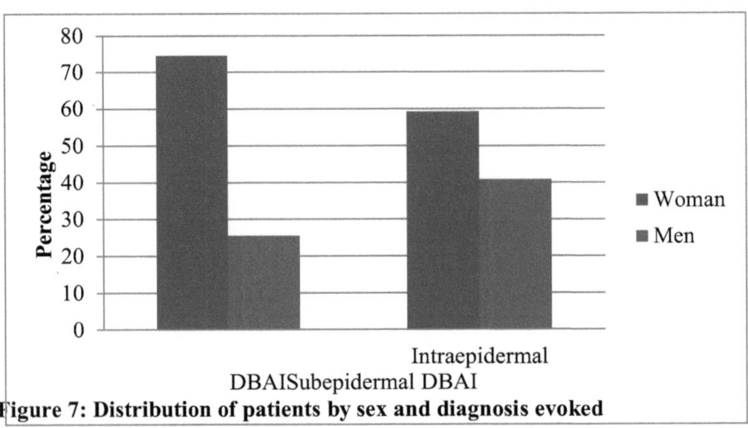

Figure 7: Distribution of patients by sex and diagnosis evoked

1.2. Clinical signs

The distribution of clinical signs observed is shown **in figure 8.** The most frequent clinical signs were pruritus (47%), bullae (38%) and erosions (22%). Lesions were associated with each other in 21% of cases.

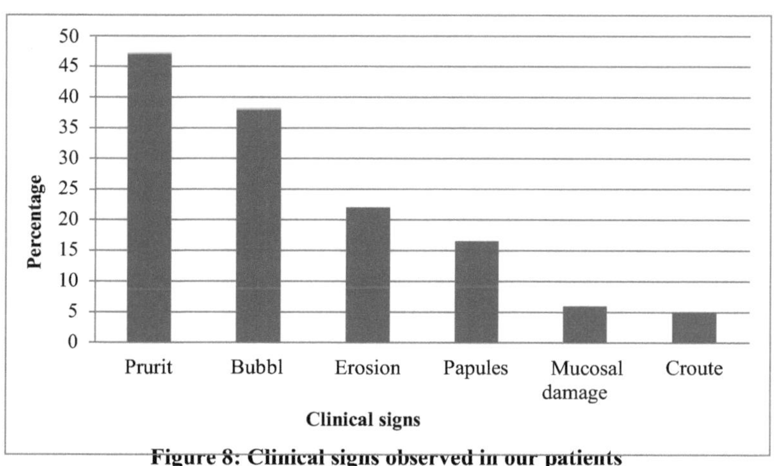

Figure 8: Clinical signs observed in our patients

1.3. Suspected clinical diagnoses

Analysis of clinical information revealed that: **(Figure 9)**

-Two hundred and forty patients (72%) were referred for suspected **subepidermal DBAI** (pemphigoid group), including several pathologies: bullous pemphigoid, cicatricial pemphigoid, pemphigoid gestationis, dermatitis herpetiformis, linear IgA dermatosis and epidermolysis bullosa acquisitiva.

-Ninety-four patients (28%) were referred for suspected **intra-epidermal DBAI** (pemphigus group): superficial pemphigus, pemphigus vulgaris, paraneoplastic pemphigus, pemphigus herpetiformis, pemphigus vegetans.

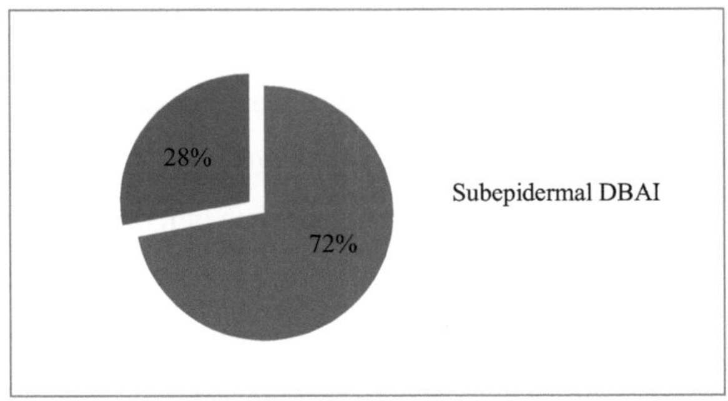

Figure 9: Distribution of suspected clinical diagnoses in included patients

The distribution of clinical signs according to the diagnosis evoked is shown in **Table I**. Pruritus and bullae were the most frequent signs in sub-epidermal DBAI, with frequencies of 59% and 40% respectively, while erosions were most frequently observed (49%) in patients with suspected intra-epidermal DBAI.

Table I: Distribution of clinical signs according to the diagnosis evoked

	Subepidermal DBAI (n= 240)		**Intraepidermal DBAI (n= 94)**	
		N%		**N%**
Pruritus	141	**59**	17	18
Croute	10	4	8	8,5
Erosion	28	12	46	**49**
Bubble	96	**40**	30	32
Papule	41	17	14	15
Mucosal damage	7	3	14	15

1.4. Direct immunofluorescence results

IFD was negative in 56% of cases and positive in 44% (**Figure 10**).

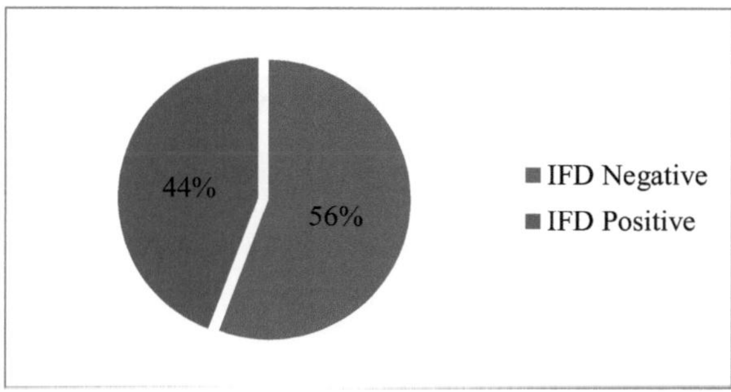

Figure 10: IFD results in our series

1.4.1. Negative IFD

A negative IFD, defined as the absence of Ig and complement deposits in the skin, was observed in 186 cases, i.e. 56% of the total number of cases studied.

IFD was negative in 46 cases of pemphigus (49%) and in 140 cases of pemphigoid (58%).

1.4.2. Positive IFD

A positive DTI, indicating the presence of Ig and/or complement deposits in the skin, was noted in 148 cases, or 44% of all cases studied.

The IFD was positive in 48 cases of pemphigus (51%) and in 100 cases of pemphigus.

pemphigoid (42%).

1.4.2.1. Type of deposit

The various deposits observed are illustrated in **figure 11**. C3 and IgG deposits were the most frequently observed (92% and 28% respectively), while IgA deposits were the least frequent (10%).

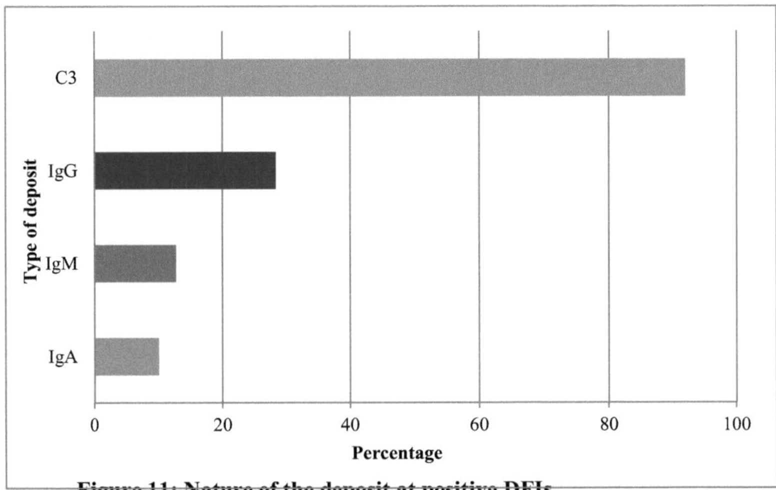

Figure 11: Nature of the deposit at positive DFIs

-For subepidermal DBAI, isolated C3 deposits were the most frequently observed, accounting for around 2/3 of cases. C3 deposits associated with IgG were observed in 11% of cases **(Figure 12)**.

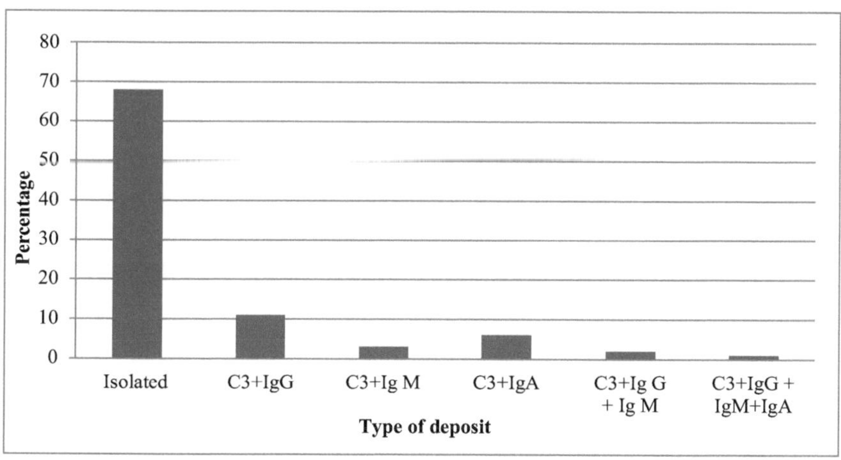

Figure 12: Different deposits observed on IFD in subepidermal DBAI

-For intra-epidermal DBAI: the most frequently observed deposit was that of IgG associated with the C3 fraction of complement (44%). An isolated C3 deposit was observed in 21% of cases, and associated with IgM in 19% **(Figure 13)**.

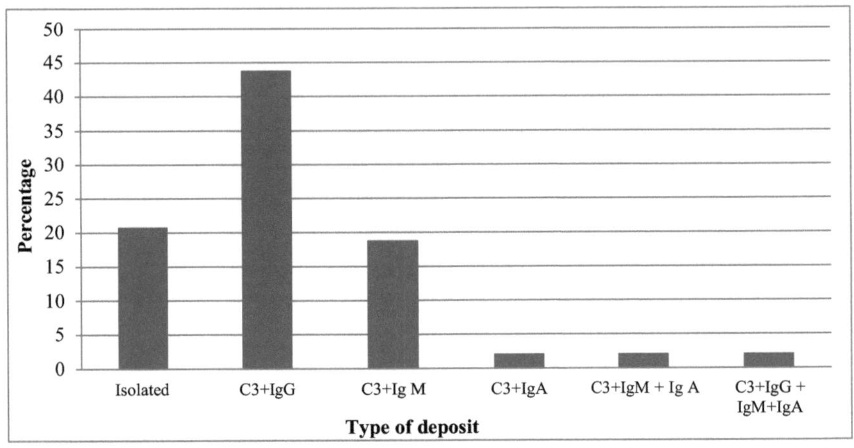

Figure 13: The different deposits observed on IFD in intra-epidermal DBAI

1.4.2.2. Deposit location and appearance

Table II illustrates the different types of deposits observed and their location.

-Localized intercellular deposition in the epidermis was observed in 40 patients (27%). In all cases, the appearance was mesh-like.

-Deposition on the EDJ was observed in 102 patients (69%). The appearance was linear in 72 patients (70.5%) and granular in 30 (29.5%).

-Four patients (3%) had a net-mesh intraepidermal deposit associated with a JDE deposit.

-Two patients (1%) had vascular deposits.

Table II: Different aspects of the deposits observed at the IFD and their location

Location	Aspect	Observation with a fluorescence microscope (X400)
Epidermis (N=40 ; 27%)	Net mesh (N=40; 100%)	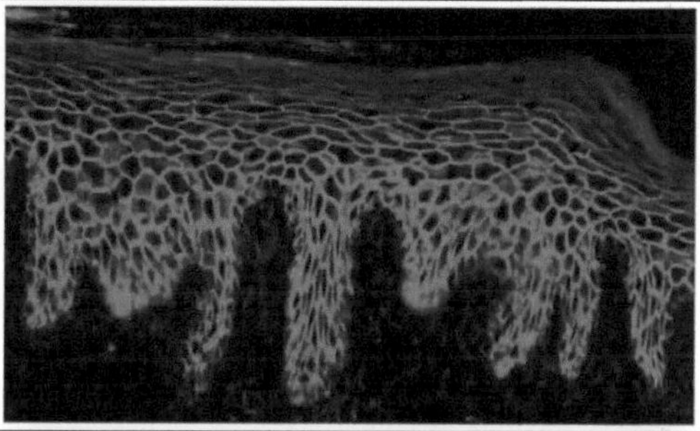
Dermal-epidermal junction (DEJ) (N=102; 69%)	Linear (N=72 ; 70,5%)	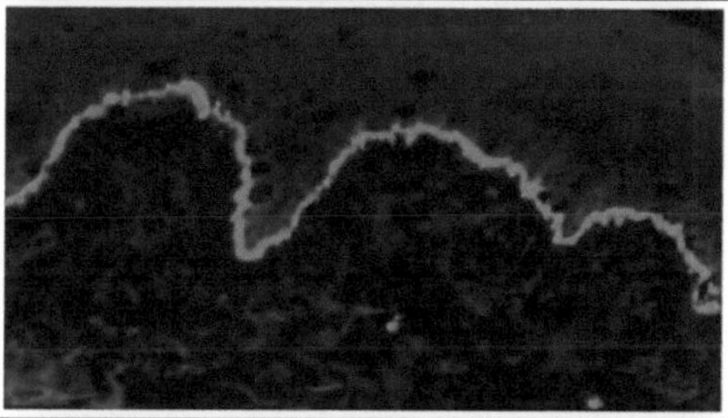
	Granular (N=30; 29.5%)	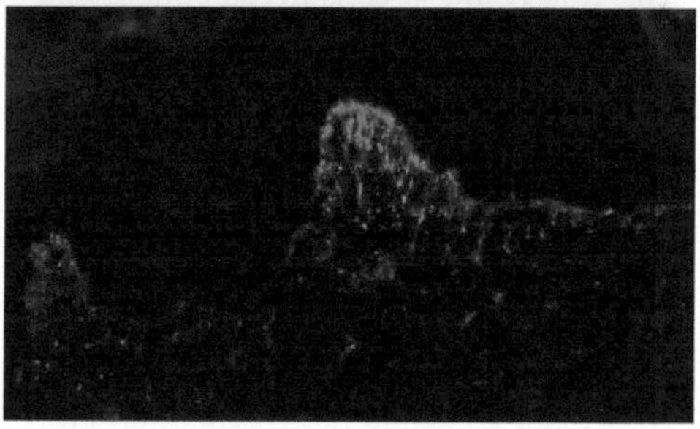

Epidermis +JDE (N=4 ; 3%)	-Mesh from net+linear (N=2 ; 50%)	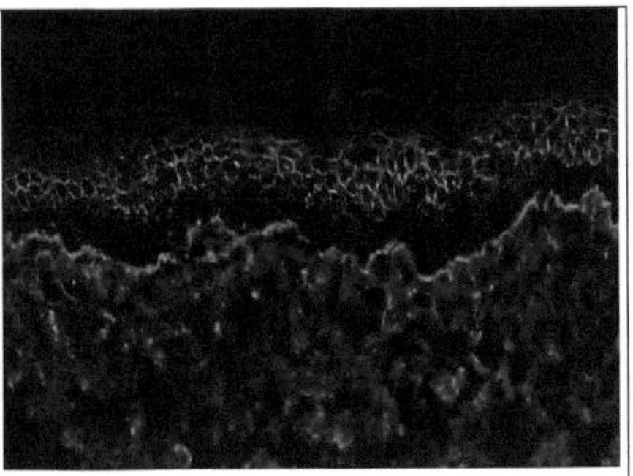
	-Mesh from net+granular (N=2 ; 50%)	

2. Analytical study

The study of the association between suspected diagnosis and IFD results is **shown in Tables III and IV**.

The IFD result is considered concordant with the clinical diagnosis if it shows a C3 deposit, with or without Ig, in the JDE in the case of sub-epidermal DBAI, and a mesh-like deposit of Ig±C3 in the epidermis in the case of intra-epidermal DBAI.

Overall, there was agreement between the DFI result and the clinical diagnosis in 90% of cases. This concordance was 93% in sub-epidermal DBAI and 87.5% in intra-epidermal DBAI.

Table III: Concordance between IFD results and clinical diagnosis

	IFD	N	%
Intra-epidermal DBAI (n=48)	Concordante	42	87,5
	Discordant	6	12,5
Subepidermal DBAI (n=100)	Concordante	93	93
	Discordant	7	7

Table IV: Summary of IFD findings by clinical diagnosis

	Deposit at JDE (N= 102)		Mesh-like deposition in the epidermis (N=40)		Deposit at JDE + epidermis (N=4)		Vascular deposit (N=2)		Total
	N	%	N	%	N	%	N	%	
DBAIintra	7	14,6	37	77	4	8,4	0	0	48
DBAIsous	95	95	3	3	0	0	2	2	100

Discussion

Autoimmune bullous dermatoses (ABD) are a heterogeneous group of diseases with variable prognosis. They are organ-specific AIDs linked to the production of auto-Ac directed against epidermal or EDD structures.

The structure of the skin is important for understanding the pathophysiology of DBAI.

1. Skin structure

The skin is made up of 3 superimposed parts **(Figure 14):**

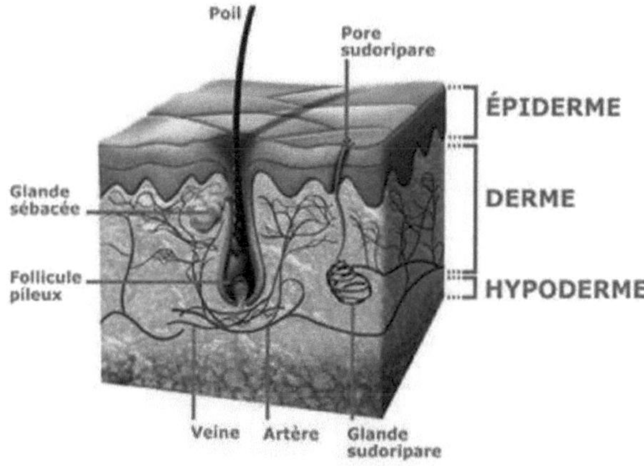

Figure 14: Ultrastructure of the skin

- **Epidermis:** the outermost layer in contact with the air, composed of stratified layers of cells, mainly keratinocytes. Cellular adhesion between two adjacent keratinocytes is ensured by **the desmosome**. The epidermis is linked to the dermis by the JDE.

  The epidermis is made up of several layers: (i) the basal layer, which is in direct contact with the JDE (basal membrane) via **hemidesmosomes**, (ii) the spinous layer, (iii) the granular layer and (iv) the clear layer and stratum corneum, the most superficial part of the epidermis **(Figure 15).**

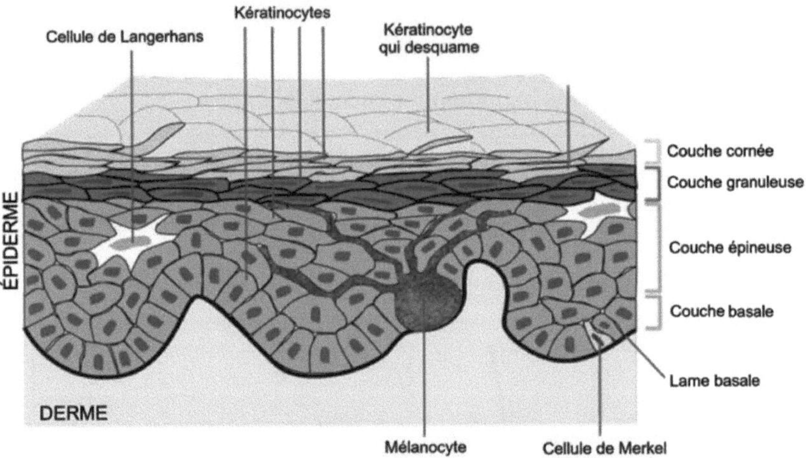

Figure 15: The different layers of the epidermis

- **Dermis:** connected to the epidermis at the basement membrane. It is composed of cells, mainly immune cells and fibroblasts, and an extracellular matrix (collagen and elastic fibers) that gives the skin its elasticity. The dermis is also home to blood vessels, nerves and glands.
- **Hypodermis:** the deepest layer of the skin (6), a loose, richly vascularized connective tissue made up mainly of adipose tissue, which acts as a protective padding, insulation and energy reservoir.

Desmosomes and hemidesmosomes are anchoring junctions that mechanically bind cells together:

- Desmosomes

Inter-keratinocyte cohesion is fundamental to the organization and maintenance of epidermal architecture and function. Together with other structures, desmosomes ensure cohesion between keratinocytes.

The desmosome is a multimolecular complex made up of transmembrane glycoproteins belonging to the desmosomal cadherin family (desmogleins (Dsg) and desmocollins (Dsc)), which form the desmoglia, and cytosolic proteins; plakins (desmoplakins (DP), plectin (PL), envoplakin (ENV) and periplakin (PPL)) and armadillo proteins (plakoglobin (PG) and plakophilins (PKP)), which form the desmosomal plate (7,8).

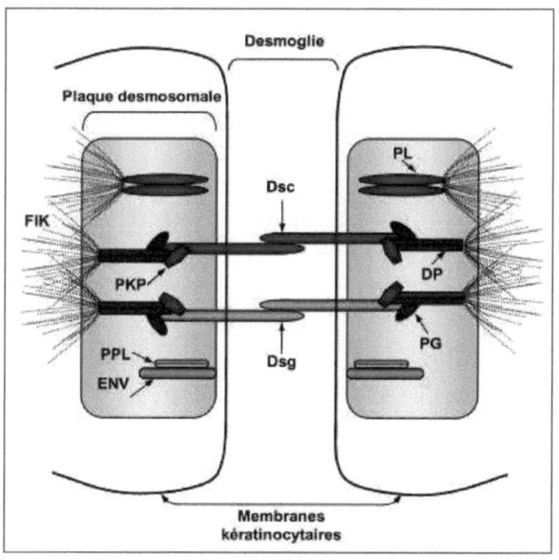

Figure 16: Molecular structure of the desmosome (8)

- **Hemidesmosomes**

The JDE forms an adhesion zone between the epidermis and the dermis. This adhesion is ensured by hemidesmosomes, anchoring filaments and anchoring fibrils. Hemidesmosome/anchoring filament complexes anchor basal keratinocytes to the basement membrane, which is made up of 2 laminae: lamina lucida and lamina densa (8,9) **(Figure 17)**.

The hemidesmosome is composed of several types of proteins: hemidesmosomal plaque proteins (BP230 also known as bullous pemphigoid antigen 1 BPAG1) and plectin), transmembrane proteins (integrin a6β4 and BP180) and basement membrane-associated proteins (laminin and type IV collagen)(8).

Figure 17: Structure of the hemidesmosome (10)

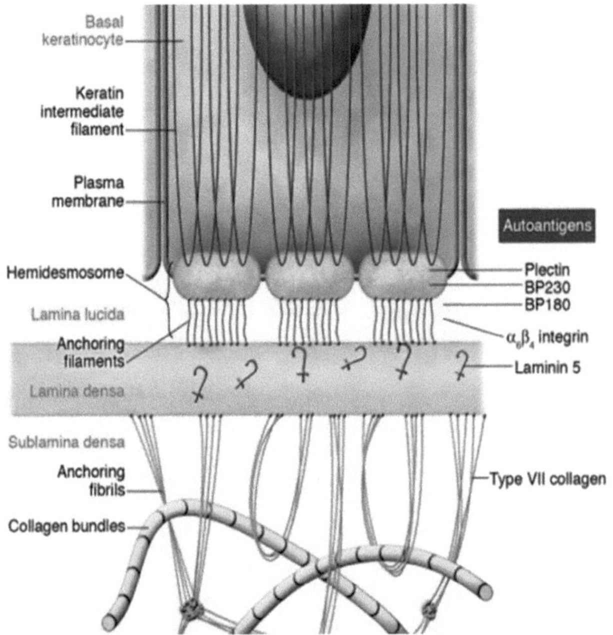

2. Autoimmune bullous dermatoses

DBAI are organ-specific autoimmune diseases characterized by the production of auto-Ac directed against structures of the epidermis or JDE junction.

These conditions have been described since the late 19th^{ème} century. But it wasn't until the 1960s that their autoimmune origin was demonstrated, thanks to the detection of anti-skin Ac in patients' serum (11).

The precise diagnosis of these diseases is based on clinical (presence of cutaneous and/or mucosal erosions and/or bullae), histopathological and immunopathological criteria (search for Ig deposition more or less associated with deposition of the C3 fraction of complement in the skin by IFD; and search for circulating anti-skin Ac by IFI or ELISA techniques).

A distinction is therefore made between:

2.1 Subepidermal DBAI

Subepidermal DBAI is characterized by loss of dermal-epidermal adhesion due to alteration of one of the components of the JDE (usually hemidesmosomes) by auto-Ac. Subepidermal DBAI comprises several entities **(Table V).**

-Epidemiologically, most authors have reported a predominance of the disease in patients aged over 70 (13,17,18). Our results are consistent with this literature.

-Clinically, the picture is dominated by pruritus and bullae. The latter are tense and often large, with clear contents (11).

Table V: Autoimmune bullous dermatoses (ABD)

Intraepidermal DBAI	Subepidermal DBAI
- Pemphigus vulgaris	-Bullous pemphigoid
-Pemphigus vegetans	-Scarring pemphigoid
-Pemphigus foliaceae (including pemphigus erythematous)	-Gestational pemphigoid
	-Linear IgA bullous dermatosis
-Pemphigus herpetiformis	-Dermatitis herpetiformis
-Paraneoplastic pemphigus	-Epidermolysis bullosa acquisita
-IgA pemphigus	
- Induced pemphigus	

2.2 Intraepidermal DBAI

Intraepidermal DBAI (or the pemphigus group) is characterized byloss of keratinocyte cohesion due to alteration of desmosomes by auto-Ac. The pemphigus group comprises various entities **(Table V).**

-Epidemiologically, a female predominance of the disease has been reported in most studies (12-15). Our series is consistent in terms of sex ratio. Indeed, pemphigus of southern Tunisia is a world-renowned entity characterized by the predominance of pemphigus erythematosus in young women, often of rural origin (16).

-Clinically, intraepidermal DBAI is characterized by fleeting intraepidermal bullae. Due to their fragility, these bullae are easily ruptured, giving way to painful erosions (11).

In our study, we conducted a retrospective descriptive study to investigate the results observed with IFD in order to assess the contribution of this technique in the diagnosis of DBAI.

3. The value of IFD in diagnosing DBAI

IFD, a one-step labeling technique, enables the detection of Ig deposits (IgG, IgA or IgM) and/or complement fractions (C3) in tissues using polyclonal Ac (anti-human Ig) conjugated to a fluorochrome (FITC).

The diagnostic performance of IFD is influenced by the pre-analytical conditions of the sample. To guarantee a reliable result, it is essential to ensure the quality of the skin biopsy received (sample taken from peri-lesional skin, sent without fixation and ideally before any treatment).

DFI plays an important role in the diagnosis of AIBD. It is useful for differentiating autoimmune bullous dermatoses from those of non-immunological mechanism (19).

Within the DBAI framework, 2 aspects can be observed at IFD:

-Intercellular honeycomb marking in the epithelium, which is very common in intra-epidermal DBAI.

-A linear or granular marking of the basement membrane, which is often present in subepidermal DBAI (11).

Ig deposits are generally associated with C3.

Nevertheless, IFD provides only limited information on the target antigen(s). Thus, depending on the nature of the Ig and/or complement deposit, its location and observed appearance, further investigation may be required to determine the antigenic target(s) and refine the diagnosis (2).

3.1 Subepidermal DBAI

In patients with suspected subepidermal DBAI, IFD was positive in 42% of cases. IFD results were consistent with the suspected clinical diagnosis in 93% of cases, revealing linear or granular deposition of C3 and/or Ig in the JDE. This aspect is compatible with what has been described in the literature (11).

In our series, isolated C3 deposits were the most frequently observed, accounting for 68% of cases. A C3 deposit associated with IgG was observed in 11% of cases.

In the literature, the sensitivity of DFI in subepidermal DBAI varies between 80% (cicatricial pemphigoid) and 100% (bullous pemphigoid) (20), provided the DFI technique is followed. However, this sensitivity may be altered by certain parameters:

-Age of the disease: at a very early stage of the disease, the DTI may be negative, or positive for C3 only. IgG deposits may appear on DTI after a few weeks.

-Biopsy site: the recommended site is the peribulbar skin.

- Long-term corticosteroid therapy can distort IFD interpretation.

However, the specificity of IFD is less than its sensitivity. Indeed, some sub-epidermal DBAIs (bullous pemphigoid, cicatricial pemphigoid, epidermolysis bullosa acquisita and pemphigoid gravidarum) generally give the same appearance on IFD (5,19).

Similarly, lupus can have a similar DFI. It is therefore essential to compare clinical data (age, appearance of skin lesions, evolution), biology, histology and IFD (appearance, nature and intensity of deposits).

Dermatitis herpetiformis and linear IgA dermatosis are more suggestive on IFD (IgA deposits at the top of the dermal papillae in the former case, and along the JDE in the 2ème case).

⇨ Thus, DFI is an indispensable examination for the diagnosis of subepidermal DBAI, but the data it provides remain limited for differentiating subgroups. This suggests the need to use complementary tests and to compare DFI results with clinical and histological data.

3.2 Intraepidermal DBAI

In patients with suspected intraepidermal DBAI, IFD was positive in 51% of cases. IFD results were consistent with the diagnosis of pemphigus in 87.5% of cases. The appearance observed was that of a net-like intercellular deposit of Ig ± C3 in the epidermis. This is consistent with the literature (11).

In our series, the most frequently observed deposit was IgG associated with the C3 fraction of complement (44%). Isolated C3 deposition was observed in 21%.

A positive DFI has important diagnostic value in cases of suspected pemphigus.

If IFD is performed under optimal conditions (sampling in peri-bullous skin, good preservation, etc.), its sensitivity to the state phase or active form of the disease can be between 85% and 90% (20).

Intra-epidermal DBAI essentially comprises deep pemphigus (vulgaris or vegetans), superficial pemphigus (foliaceous, erythematous, herpetiform) and rarer specific forms (paraneoplastic, induced, IgA).

IFD is generally unable to differentiate between superficial and deep forms of the disease, since the deposit is often present in both the deep and superficial layers of the epidermis. Paraneoplastic pemphigus, on the other hand, is a rare form of the disease, often associated with malignant proliferations, notably lymphoid hemopathies (15,21).

The appearance on IFD is quite suggestive, but not pathognomonic: association of intra-epidermal Ig ± C3 deposition with deposition in the JDE. We observed this appearance in 4 of our patients with suspected paraneoplastic pemphigus.

It should also be noted that a deposit made of isolated C3 fraction can be observed in many non-specific inflammatory dermatoses (11).

⇨ IFD plays a key role in the diagnosis of intra-epidermal DBAI, given its clinical and histological polymorphism, and the precocity of its positivity.

When the deposits are made up of IgG and C3 (and IgA for IgA pemphigus) in the epidermis, the appearance is strongly suggestive of pemphigus.

Figure 18 summarizes the different types of deposits and their location according to clinical diagnosis.

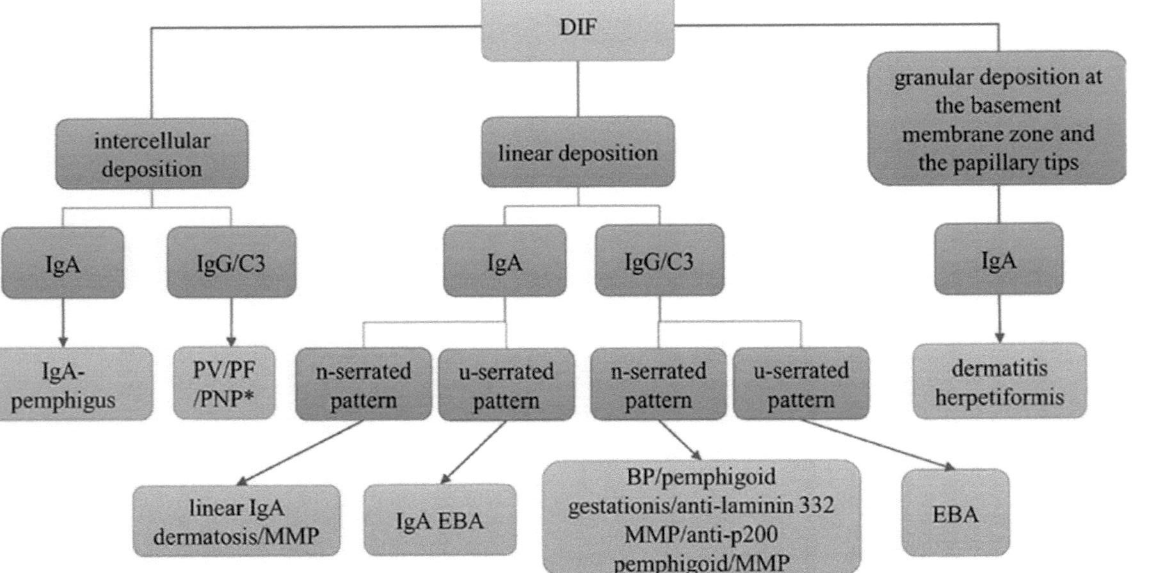

Figure 18: Summary diagram of DFI data (nature and location of deposit) in the main DBAIs

Conclusion

Autoimmune bullous dermatoses (ABD) are specific autoimmune diseases of the skin and mucous membranes. They are characterized by Ig ± complement deposition either in the epidermis, altering keratinocyte cohesion (intra-epidermal DBAI: pemphigus group), or at the dermo-epidermal junction (sub-epidermal DBAI: pemphigoid group).

The clinical presentation of DBAI is polymorphous. Diagnosis is based on clinical, histopathological and immunological criteria.

The aims of this study were to describe the results observed with direct immunofluorescence (DIF) in the different DBAIs in 1er time and to study the contribution of this technique in the diagnosis of sub- and intra-epidermal DBAIs in 2ème time.

For this fact, we conducted a retrospective descriptive study over a period from January 2018 to March 2022 covering skin biopsies received at the immunology laboratory of Habib Bourguiba Sfax University Hospital for suspected DBAI. Ig ± complement deposition was investigated by IFD using fluorochrome-conjugated polyclonal anti-human Ig Ac (IgG, IgA, IgM, C3).

We included 334 patients divided into 94 cases (28%) with suspected intraepidermal DBAI and 240 cases (72%) with suspected subepidermal DBAI. IFD was positive in 148 patients (48 cases of pemphigus and 100 cases of pemphigoid).

Our results show that :

⇨ Epidemiologically, all patients were predominantly female. Pemphigus was predominant in women aged between 40 and 49, while pemphigoid was predominant in subjects aged over 70.

⇨ Immunologically, IFD was positive in 44% of DBAI cases, with 51% in the pemphigus group and 42% in the pemphigoid group. There was agreement between the IFD result and the suspected clinical diagnosis in 90% of cases.

In cases of suspected subepidermal DBAI, DFI results were consistent with the suspected clinical diagnosis in 93% of cases, revealing linear or granular deposition of C3 and/or Ig in the EDJ.
In cases of suspected intraepidermal DBAI, IFD results were consistent with the diagnosis of pemphigus in 87.5% of cases. The most frequently observed appearance was that of a net-like intercellular deposit of Ig ± C3 in the epidermis.

Our results confirm that DFI has an important place in the diagnosis of DBAI, enabling differentiation between intra-epidermal and sub-epidermal DBAI. However, the data it provides remain limited for differentiating most subgroups of sub- and intra-epidermal DBAI. Thus, DFI data must always be compared with clinical and histological data, in order to better orientate other complementary examinations.

References

1. Bonnotte B. Pathogenic mechanisms of autoimmune diseases. Vol. 25, Revue de Medecine Interne. Elsevier Masson SAS; 2004. p. 648-58.

2. Witte M, Zillikens D, Schmidt E. Diagnosis of Autoimmune Blistering Diseases. Front Med. 2018;5:296.

3. Hofmann SC, Juratli HA, Eming R. Bullous autoimmune dermatoses. JDDG J der Dtsch Dermatologischen Gesellschaft. 2018;16(11):1339-58.

4. Sinha P, Sandhu S, Bhatia JK, Anand N, Yadav AK. Analysis of the utility of direct immunofluorescence in the diagnosis of common immune mediated dermatological conditions. J Mar Med Soc. 2020;22(1):44.

5. Menzinger S, Frassati-Biaggi A, Fraitag S, Leclerc-Mercier S. Direct immunofluorescence in dermatology: main indications. Rev Francoph des Lab. 2019;2019(508):48–55.

6. Yousef H, Alhajj M, Sharma S. Anatomy, Skin , Epidermis. 2022.

7. Emily Joo E, Yamada KM. Cell Adhesion and Movement. Stem Cell Biol Tissue Eng Dent Sci. 2015;61-72.

8. Mouquet H. Le Role De L ' Autoantigene Dans Les Maladies Auto-Immunes: Etude De La Desmogleine 1 Au Cours Des Pemphigus Le Role De L ' Autoantigene Dans Les Maladies Auto-Immunes: Etude De La Desmogleine 1 Au Cours Des Pemphigus. 2006;100.

9. Borradori L, Sonnenberg A. Structure and Function of Hemidesmosomes: More Than Simple Adhesion Complexes. J Invest Dermatol. 1999;112(4):411-8.

10. Hertl M, Eming R, Veldman C. T cell control in autoimmune bullous skin disorders. J Clin Invest. 2006;116(5):1159-66.

11. Humbel L. Autoantibodies and autoantigens in the skin. J Am Acad Dermatol.

12. Marazza G, Pham HC, Schärer L, Pedrazzetti PP, Hunziker T, Trüeb RM, et al. Incidence of bullous pemphigoid and pemphigus in Switzerland: A 2-year prospective study. Br J Dermatol. 2009;161(4):861-8.

13. Alpsoy E, Akman-Karakas A, Uzun S. Geographic variations in epidemiology of two autoimmune bullous diseases: pemphigus and bullous pemphigoid. Arch Dermatol Res. 2015 May 1;307(4):291-8.

14. Zaraa I, Kerkeni N, Ishak F, Zribi H, El Euch D, Mokni M, et al. Spectrum of autoimmune blistering dermatoses in Tunisia: An 11-year study and a review of the literature. Int J Dermatol. 2011;50(8):939-44.

15. Basu K, Chatterjee M, De A, Sengupta M, Datta C, Mitra P. A Clinicopathological and Immunofluorescence Study of Intraepidermal Immunobullous Diseases. Indian J Dermatol. 2019;64(2):101.

16. Bastuji-Garin S, Turki H, Mokhtar I, Nouira R, Fazaa B, Jomaa B, et al.Possible relation of tunisian pemphigus with traditional cosmetics: A multicenter case-control study. Am J Epidemiol. 2002;155(3):249-56.

17. Heng LC, Phoon YW, Pang SM, Lee HY. Pemphigoid and pemphigus: Comparative analysis of clinical epidemiology, course and outcome in an Asian Academic Medical Centre. Australas J Dermatol. 2021.62(2):e288-90.

18. Buch AC, Kumar H, Panicker NK, Misal S, Sharma YK, Gore CR. A Cross-sectional Study of Direct Immunofluorescence in the Diagnosis of Immunobullous Dermatoses. Indian J Dermatol. 2014;59(4):364.

19. Diercks GF, Pas HH, Jonkman MF. Immunofluorescence of Autoimmune Bullous Diseases. Surg Pathol Clin. 2017;10(2):505-12. 20. Ghohestani RF, Novotney J, Chaudhary M, Agah RS. Bullous Pemphigoid: From the. 2001

21. Tull TJ, Benton E. Immunobullous disease. Clin Med. 2021.21(3):162.

Summary :

Autoimmune bullous dermatoses (ABD) are specific autoimmune diseases of the skin and mucous membranes. They are characterized by Ig ± complement deposition either in the epidermis, altering keratinocyte cohesion (intra-epidermal DBAI), or at the dermo-epidermal junction (sub-epidermal DBAI).

Our aim was to describe the results observed with direct immunofluorescence (DIF) in the various DBAIs in 1er time and to study the contribution of this technique in the diagnosis of DBAIs in 2ème time.

We conducted a retrospective descriptive study over a period from January 2018 to March 2022 of skin biopsies received at the immunology laboratory of CHU Habib Bourguiba Sfax for suspected DBAI (n=334).

In cases of suspected subepidermal DBAI, IFD was positive in 42% of cases. IFD results were consistent with the suspected clinical diagnosis in 93% of cases, revealing linear or granular deposition of C3 and/or Ig in the JDE.

In cases of suspected intraepidermal DBAI, IFD was positive in 51% of cases. IFD results were consistent with the diagnosis of pemphigus in 87.5% of cases. The most frequently observed appearance was that of a net-like intercellular deposit of Ig ± C3 in the epidermis.

Our results confirm that DFI plays an important role in the diagnosis of DBAI, differentiating between intra-epidermal and sub-epidermal DBAI. The nature and location of the deposit guide other investigations to determine the antigenic target(s) and further refine the diagnosis.

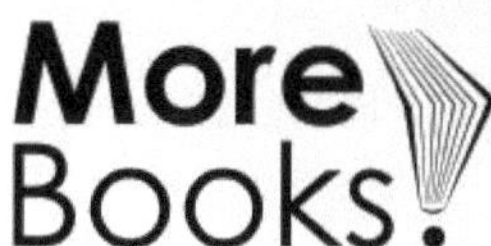

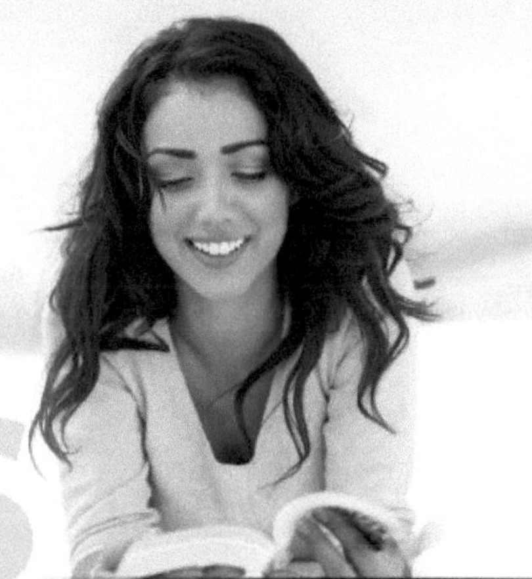

yes

I want morebooks!

Buy your books fast and straightforward online - at one of world's fastest growing online book stores! Environmentally sound due to Print-on-Demand technologies.

Buy your books online at

www.morebooks.shop

Kaufen Sie Ihre Bücher schnell und unkompliziert online – auf einer der am schnellsten wachsenden Buchhandelsplattformen weltweit! Dank Print-On-Demand umwelt- und ressourcenschonend produzi ert.

Bücher schneller online kaufen

www.morebooks.shop

info@omniscriptum.com
www.omniscriptum.com

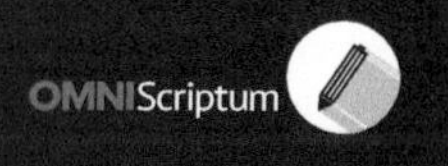

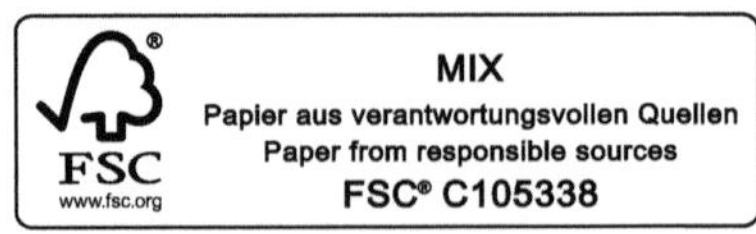

Printed by Books on Demand GmbH, Norderstedt / Germany